The Gerd Friendly Recipe Book

Discover Many Recipes that are Gut-Friendly and Absolutely Delicious!

BY: Allie Allen

COOK & ENJOY

Copyright 2020 Allie Allen

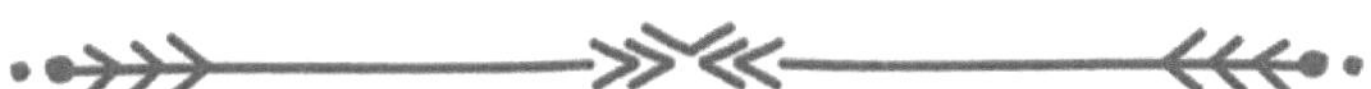

Copyright Notes

This book is written as an informational tool. While the author has taken every precaution to ensure the accuracy of the information provided therein, the reader is warned that they assume all risk when following the content. The author will not be held responsible for any damages that may occur as a result of the readers' actions.

The author does not give permission to reproduce this book in any form, including but not limited to: print, social media posts, electronic copies or photocopies, unless permission is expressly given in writing.

Table of Contents

Introduction

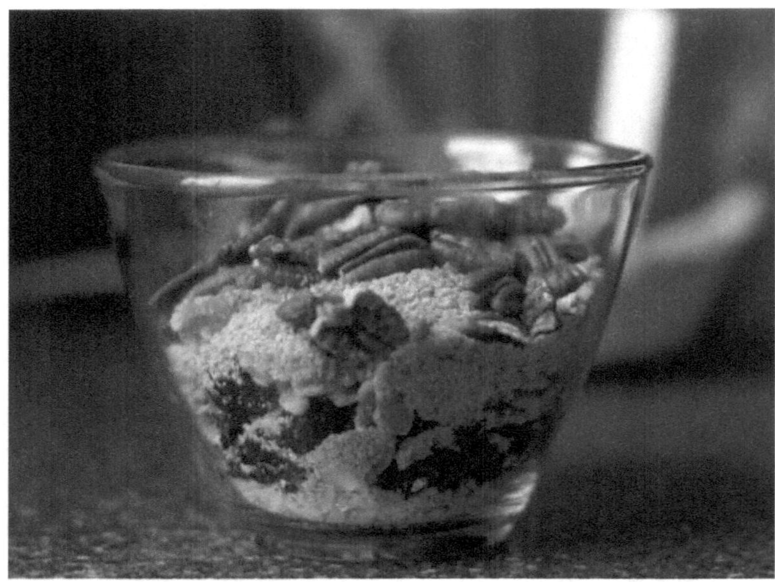

If you're looking for recipes that are delicious and good for your gut, you've come to the right place! With the help of this recipe book, you'll be able to put up 30 delicious recipes that are GERD friendly and help reduce inflammation in your gut. Plus, there's a variety of recipes in here which makes it perfect for everyone and every occasion!

All of the recipes in here are detailed and come with step-by-step instructions and so anyone can whip them up! So choose a recipe and let's begin!

Blueberry & Matcha Oatmeal

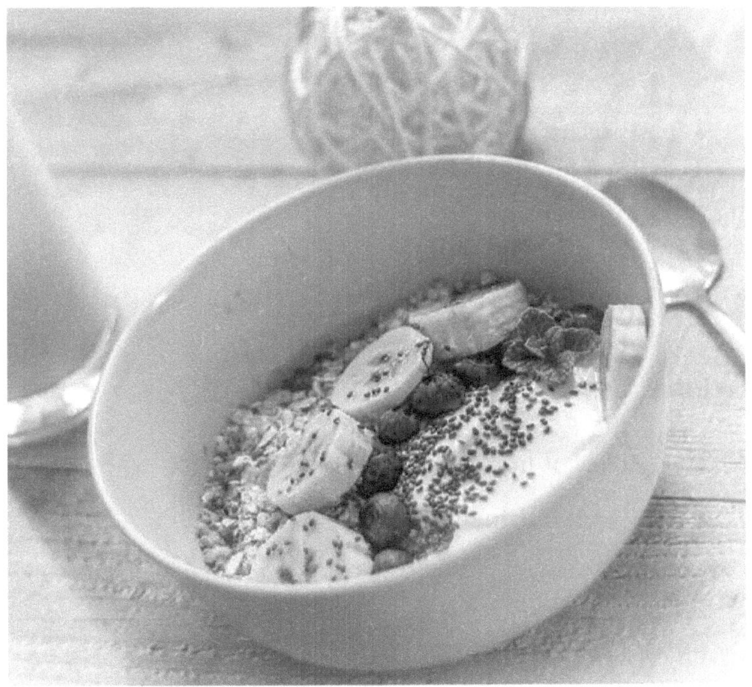

Chia seeds offer fiber-rich options for breakfast, and oatmeal is a favorite food for your gut. The combination of hemp seeds, matcha and blueberries make this a superfood breakfast.

Makes: 2 servings

Prep: 5 mins

Cook: 5 mins

Ingredients:

- 1 cup of oats, rolled
- 1 & 1/2 cups of milk, almond
- 1 scoop of collagen peptides
- 1 tbsp. of chia seeds
- 2 tbsp. of syrup, maple
- 1 tsp. of vanilla, pure
- 1/2 to 1 tsp. of matcha

To top:

- 2 tbsp. of hemp seeds
- 1/2 cup of blueberries, fresh

Directions:

Combine the almond milk, vanilla and syrup in sauce pan. Bring to boil.

Add and stir chia seeds, matcha, collagen and rolled oats into milk mixture.

Simmer for three to five minutes, till mixture absorbs all the milk.

Divide in two bowls. Top with hemp seeds, blueberries and one more drizzle of syrup. Serve.

Pineapple Blueberry Smoothie

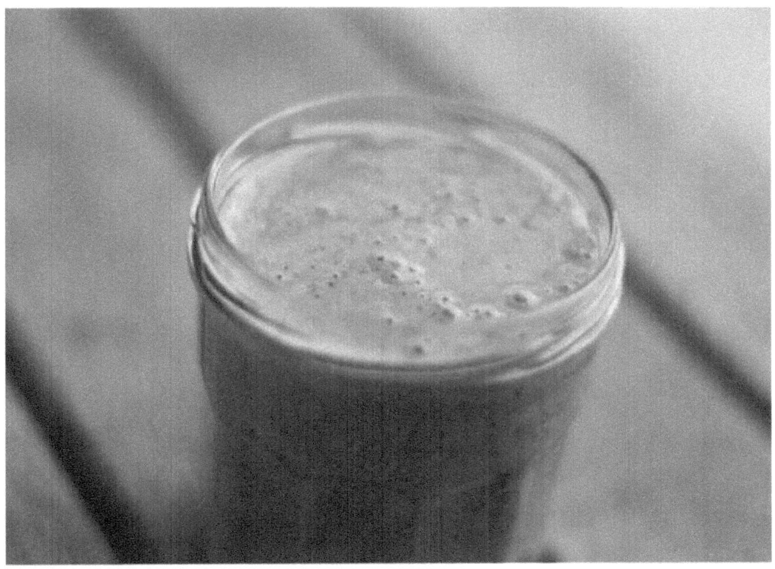

Along with whole grain quinoa flakes, tangy coconut water, healthy fat from almonds and the protein in the egg whites, this drink is a complete nutritional and delicious package.

Makes: 2 servings

Prep: 5 mins

Cook: -

Ingredients:

- 2 cups coconut water
- 1 cup pineapple chunks
- 1/3 cup quinoa flakes
- 1/2 cup pasteurized egg whites
- 1/4 cup unsalted raw or roasted almonds
- 1 tsp. vanilla extract or 1/2 tsp. almond extract
- 1/4 tsp. ground cloves
- 1 cup frozen blueberries

Directions:

Blend all the ingredients until smooth, about 30 seconds.

Divide between two glasses and serve.

Banana Walnut Oatmeal

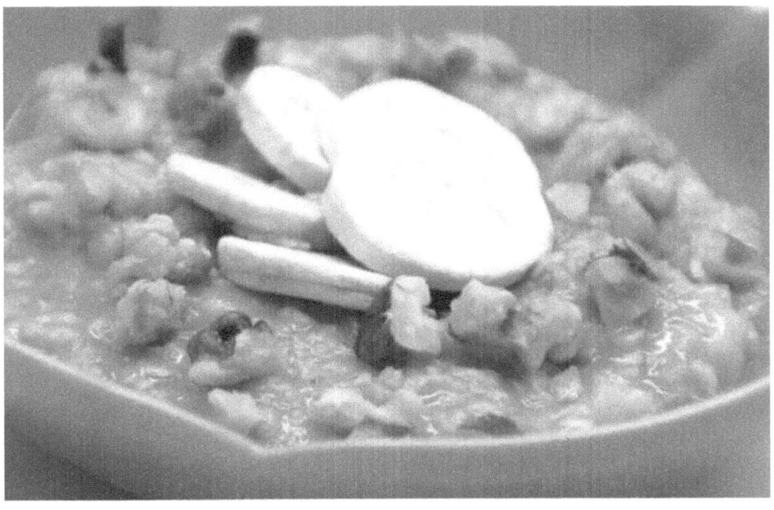

Simple, healthy and delicious banana walnut oatmeal that almost tastes like banana bread.

Makes: 2 servings

Prep: 2 mins

Cook: 5 mins

Ingredients:

- 1 cup quick-cooking oats
- 2 1/2 cups milk
- 1 tsp vanilla extract
- 2 small (or 1 large) ripe bananas, sliced
- 3 tbsp. walnuts, chopped plus extra for topping
- Honey, for topping (optional)

Directions:

In a medium-sized saucepan, combine oats, milk, vanilla extract and bananas over medium-high heat. Bring mixture to a boil, lower heat and cook for 5 minutes.

Remove pan from heat. Add in the walnuts and stir to combine.

Divide between bowls and top with more walnuts and honey, if desired.

Serve.

Chia, Spinach & Kale Muffins

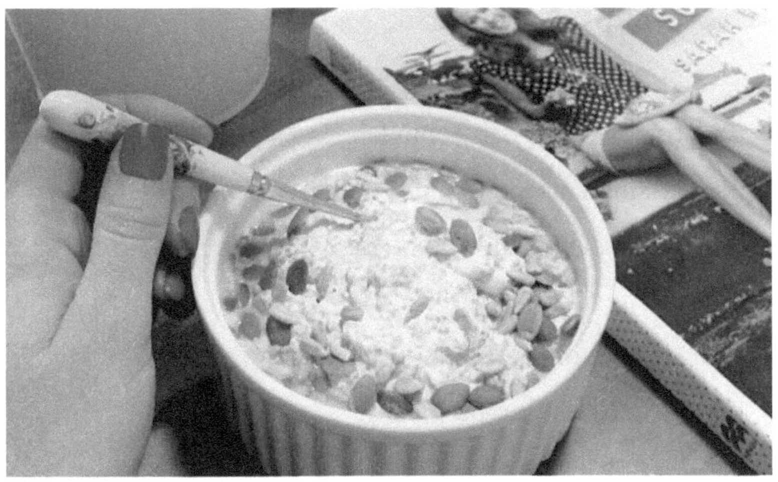

This savory breakfast is full of protein and superfoods. The muffins help in keeping your appetite at bay for the entire morning. When you top the muffins with micro greens, smashed avocados, matcha salt and quinoa, you're adding complete proteins that contain amino acids your body uses for repair and growth.

Makes: 6 servings

Prep: 10 mins

Cook: 45 mins

Ingredients:

- 3 & 1/2 ounces of sliced kale
- 2 tbsp. of oil, olive
- 1/2 tsp. of salt, sea
- 2 ounces of baby spinach leaves
- 1 small sized bunch of chives, chopped
- 2 cups of quinoa, cooked
- 3 eggs, large
- 1 tbsp. of flax seeds or chia seeds
- 2 cups of almond meal
- 2 smashed avocados
- 2 tbsp. of lemon juice, fresh
- 1 pinch salt, sea
- 2 tbsp. oil, olive
- 1 handful micro greens or sprouts

Directions:

Preheat oven to 360F.

Use oil and salt to massage leaves of kale for about three to four minutes, till they have softened.

Add the cooked quinoa, baby spinach and chives.

Beat eggs in separate bowl. Add chia seeds to that bowl.

Pour egg mixture over greens. Add almond meal, too. Mix till all is combined well.

Spoon batter into lined muffin tin cups. Bake for 35-40 minutes, till golden and cooked through.

Add lime juice and 2 tbsp. oil to smashed avocados. Pile over muffin tops.

Use micro herbs or sprouts to garnish. Serve.

Very Berry Parfait Pudding

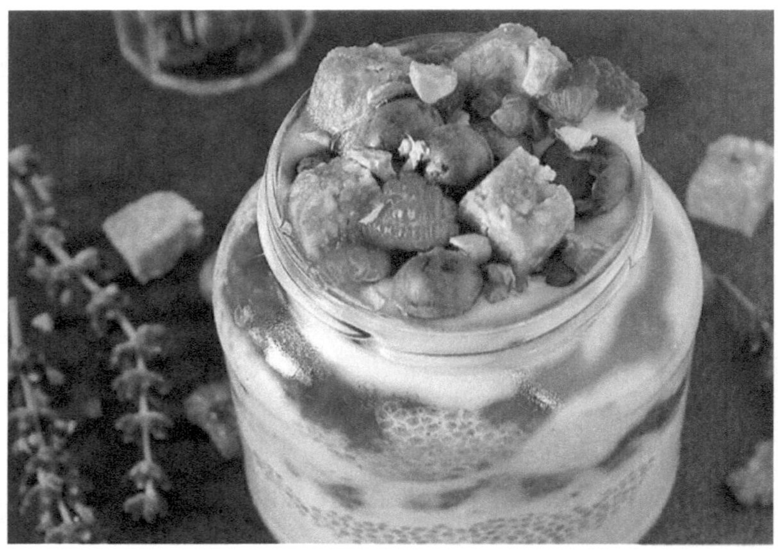

Here's a simple yet classy snack that includes yogurt and berries.

Makes: 4 servings

Prep: 10 mins

Cook: -

Ingredients:

- 2 cups fresh or frozen and thawed mixed berries such as blueberries, raspberries, and currants
- 10 ounces soft tofu (about 1 container)
- 2 tbsp. honey or agave syrup
- 1 tsp. grated orange zest or lemon zest
- 1/2 tsp. almond extract
- 1 1/2 cups plain, low-fat yogurt
- 2 tsp. vanilla extract
- 1 cup granola of choice

Directions:

Place the berries, tofu, sweetener, citrus zest, and almond extract in a blender or food processor container and blend until smooth.

In a bowl, combine the yogurt and vanilla extract.

To assemble a parfait, place some of the granola on the bottom of a parfait or other glass of choice and top with the yogurt followed by the berry pudding. Repeat so you have two layers of each.

Yogurt & Coconut Breakfast Parfait

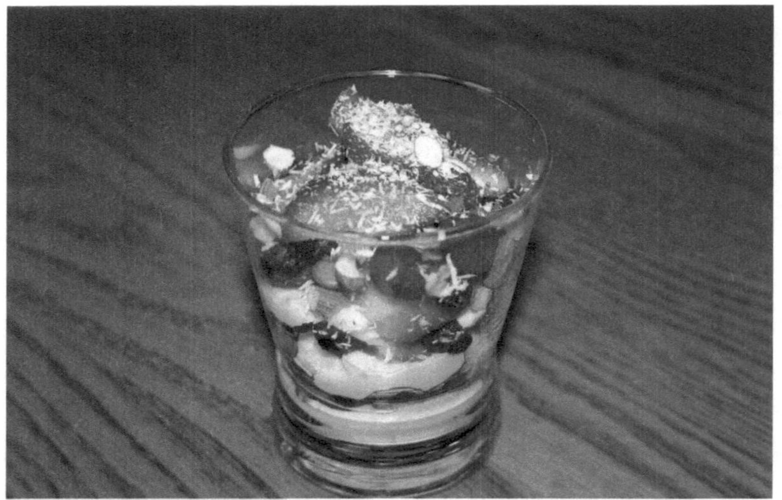

There are several things you want to look for in your breakfast – it needs to have great taste, it should keep you full for the morning, be healthy for you, and it should be easy to prepare. This parfait fills that bill and it's a delicious way to start your day.

Makes: 1 serving

Prep: 5 mins

Cook: -

Ingredients:

- 1 cup of yogurt, Greek

- 2 tbsp. of sunflower seeds

- Optional: 2 tbsp. of coconut, shredded

- A dash of cinnamon, ground

- 1/4 cup of berries, your choice of type

Optional: 1 tsp. Stevia, as desired

Directions:

Add 1/2 cup yogurt to glass or bowl.

Top yogurt with 1/8 cup of berries, cinnamon, coconut and 1 tbsp. of sunflower seeds.

Top that with remaining 1/2 cup of Greek yogurt, remaining 1/8 cup of berries, cinnamon, coconut and 1 tbsp. of sunflower seeds.

Top with Stevia if desired. Serve.

Lemon Roasted Asparagus

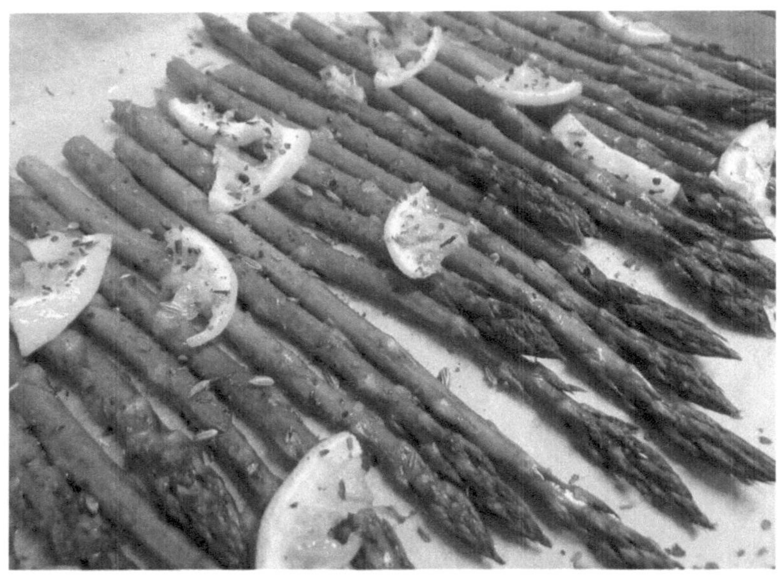

This lemony roasted asparagus with parmesan is the perfect recipe for a classic side dish that's light on your stomach.

Makes: 8 servings

Prep: 10 mins

Cook: 10 mins

Ingredients:

- 2 lb. fresh asparagus, trimmed
- ¼ cup olive oil
- 4 tbsp. Parmesan, grated
- 2 lemons, thinly sliced
- 4 tbsp. freshly squeezed lemon juice
- 1 tsp sea salt
- ½ tsp ground black pepper

Directions:

Preheat oven to 400°F. Prepare a baking sheet with baking paper.

Add all of the ingredients onto the baking sheet and toss to evenly coat. Place in the oven for about 10-15 minutes or until the asparagus is roasted.

Serve.

Labneh Summer Salad

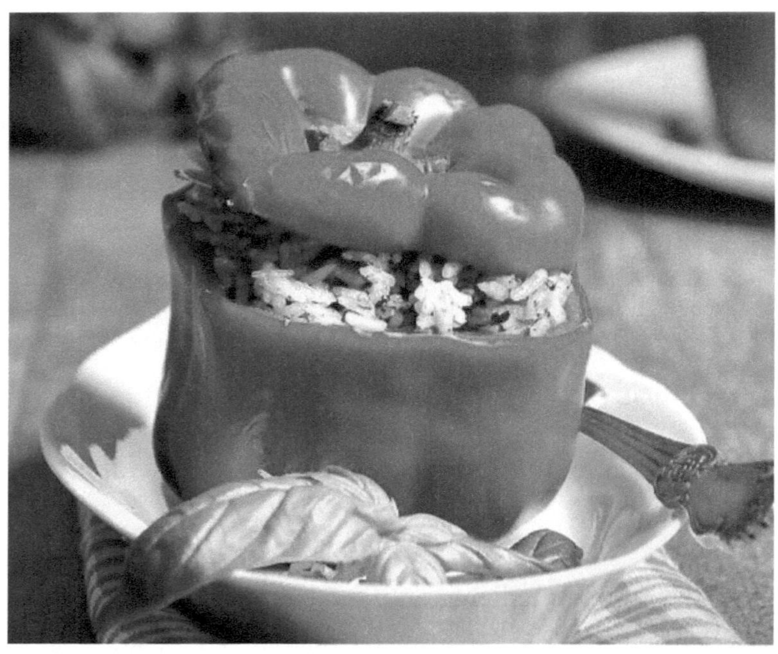

This is a fresh salad that's great for outdoor entertaining and can be served individually or family style.

Makes: 4 servings

Prep: 10 mins

Cook: -

Ingredients:

- ½ cup (120 g) labneh
- 4 cups (80 g) frisée or mixed greens of choice
- 2 cups (300 g) halved heirloom cherry tomatoes
- 2 avocados, halved and sliced
- 4 tbsp. extra-virgin olive oil, divided
- Salt and pepper, to taste
- 2 tbsp. (8 g) nigella seeds
- 1 tsp sumac
- Seeds from 1 pomegranate (optional)
- 2–3 fresh mint leaves
- Pita chips or lavash bread, for serving

Directions:

With a tbsp., scoop the labneh and smear along the bottom of four serving plates. Arrange the frisée over the labneh. Place the tomatoes in between the avocado slices. Sprinkle with 3 tbsp. of the olive oil, salt, pepper, nigella seeds, sumac and pomegranate seeds (if using). Add the mint leaves and finish with a light drizzle of the remaining 1 tbsp. olive oil.

Serve with pita chips or lavash bread.

Labneh

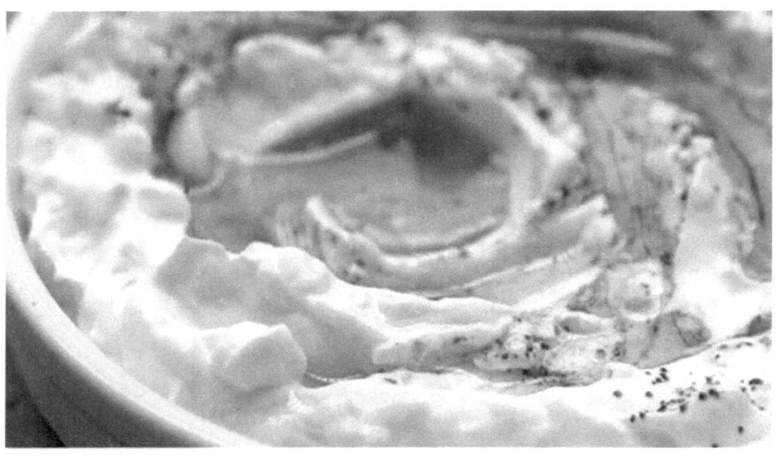

Labneh is easy to make and easy on your stomach and is delicious drizzled with good-quality olive oil and sprinkled with sea salt and herbs.

Makes: 4 servings

Prep: 4 hrs. 5 mins

Cook: -

Ingredients:

- 2 cups Greek-style plain yogurt
- ½ tsp. sea salt flakes

Directions:

Line a strainer with damp cheesecloth or a clean dish towel, then place it over a bowl. Mix the yogurt with the salt and put it into the prepared strainer. Bring the edges of the cloth up and gently twist them together to enclose the yogurt into a ball. You don't need to twist it tightly—just enough to hold the yogurt mix firmly. Secure the twist with a rubber band.

Let the yogurt drain for 4 hours; it should have the consistency of thick cream cheese. You can keep labneh in the refrigerator, covered, for up to two days.

Salmon & Avocado Dip

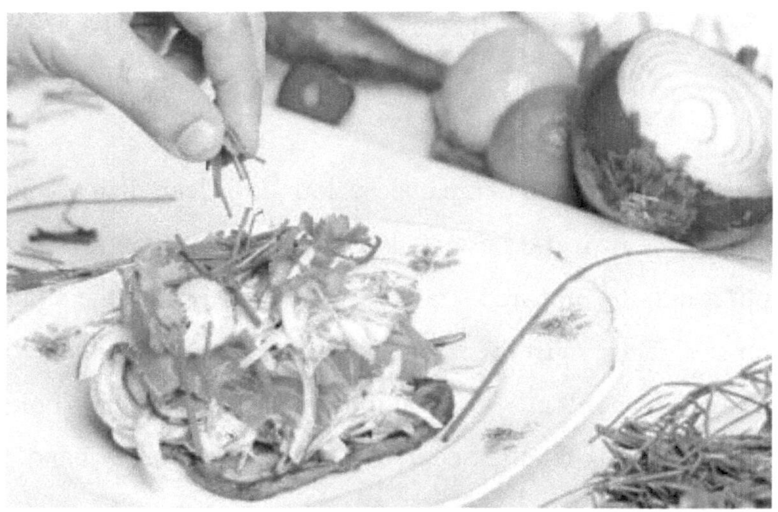

This avocado dip works so well with salmon, especially when the salmon is grilled. It's usually served with rice, as well.

Makes: 6 servings

Prep: 5 mins

Cook: 15 mins

Ingredients:

- 2 peeled, then pitted and diced avocados
- 3 tbsp. of yogurt, Greek-style
- 1 tbsp. of lemon juice, fresh
- Kosher salt & ground pepper, as desired
- 2 lbs. of salmon steaks
- 2 tsp. of dill weed, dried
- 2 tsp. of pepper, lemon

Directions:

Preheat grill for a high heat level. Oil grate lightly.

Mash avocados, lemon juice, and yogurt together in medium sized bowl. Season as desired.

Rub the salmon with lemon pepper, salt and dill. Place on grill. Cook for 15 minutes and turn once till you can flake it easily using a fork. Serve with avocado mixture.

Strawberry Cranberry Banana Smoothie

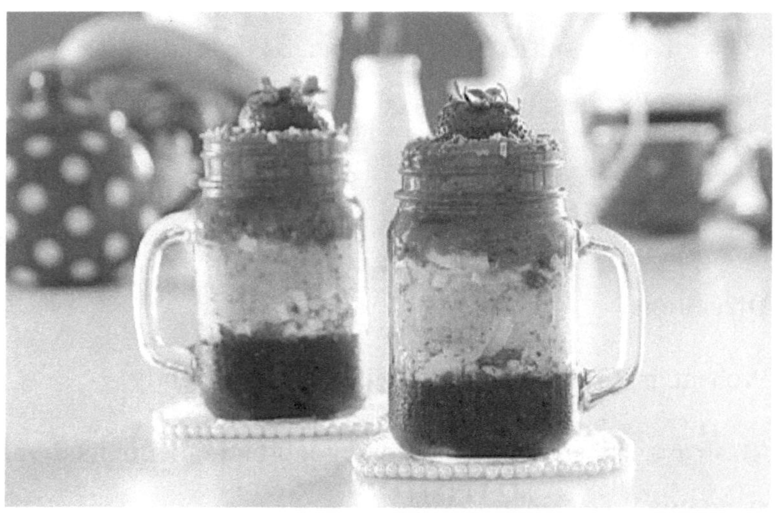

A thick, fresh and delicious smoothie that works great for breakfast and dessert.

Makes: 2 servings

Prep: 5 mins

Cook: -

Ingredients:

- 1 ½ cup strawberries
- 2 bananas
- 3 cups fresh cranberry juice

Directions:

Blend strawberries, bananas, and cranberry juice in a blender until smooth. Divide between two large glasses and serve.

Cooling Cucumber Avocado Soup

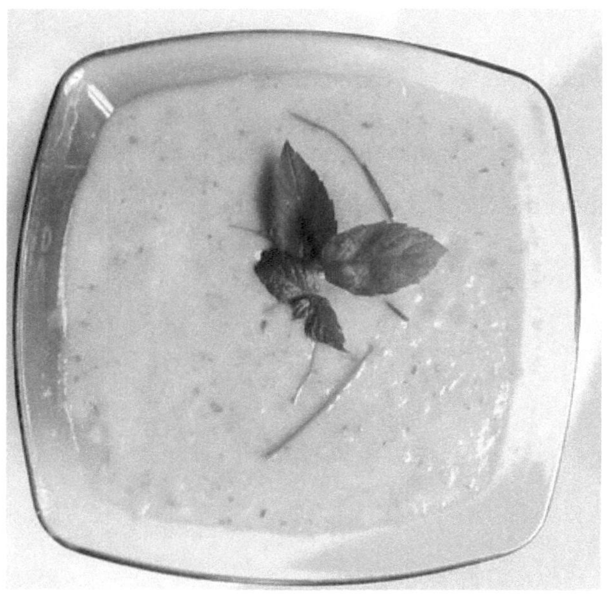

This cooling cucumber and avocado soup will cool down your gut and give you all the nutrients.

Makes: 6 servings

Prep: 15 mins + cooling time

Cook: -

Ingredients:

- 2 cups water

- 2 ripe avocados, pitted and peeled

- 1 tbsp. finely chopped fresh cilantro

- 2 lb. English cucumbers, seeded, peeled, & cut

- ¼ tsp. maple syrup

- 3 tbsp. lime juice

- Salt

- 1 tbsp. finely chopped fresh mint

Directions:

Pour just one cup of water into a blender, & then add the avocados, cucumbers, lime juice, & maple syrup, ¼ tsp. of salt. Blend till smooth. Taste & adjust seasoning.

Chill for two hrs., then stir in the mint & cilantro & serve.

Green Beans with Brazil Nuts and Basil

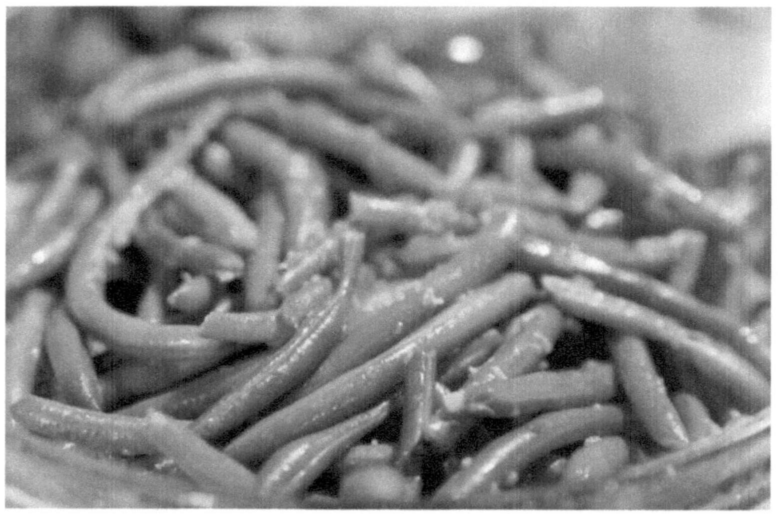

Green beans are a popular vegetable. This dish is dairy free and delicious. Plus it's topped with Brazil nuts because they're an amazing source of the mineral selenium, which some research suggests lessens chemotherapy's toxic effects on healthy hair, kidney, and GI tract cells.

Makes: 12 servings

Prep: 15 mins

Cook: 10 mins

Ingredients:

- Freshly squeezed lemon juice
- 2 pound green beans, trimmed
- 1/4 cup olive oil
- 1/4 cup finely chopped fresh basil
- Sea salt
- 1/4 cup chopped shallot
- Freshly ground pepper
- 1/4 cup finely ground Brazil nuts or walnuts
- ½ tsp. lemon zest

Directions:

Bring a good amount of water (about 16 cups) to a boil. Add 1/2 tsp of salt & the green beans & cook until tender-crisp, 6-8 mins. Drain & then run them under cold water.

Heat the 1/2 cup olive oil in a pan over med heat, & then add the shallot & a pinch of salt & sauté for about 1 minute. Add in the beans, add 1/2 tsp. of salt, & cook, until heated through, about 2 mins. Remove & add several grinds of pepper, a splash of the lemon juice, & the nuts. Toss with the basil & lemon zest before serving.

Pasta Primavera, No-Cream Style

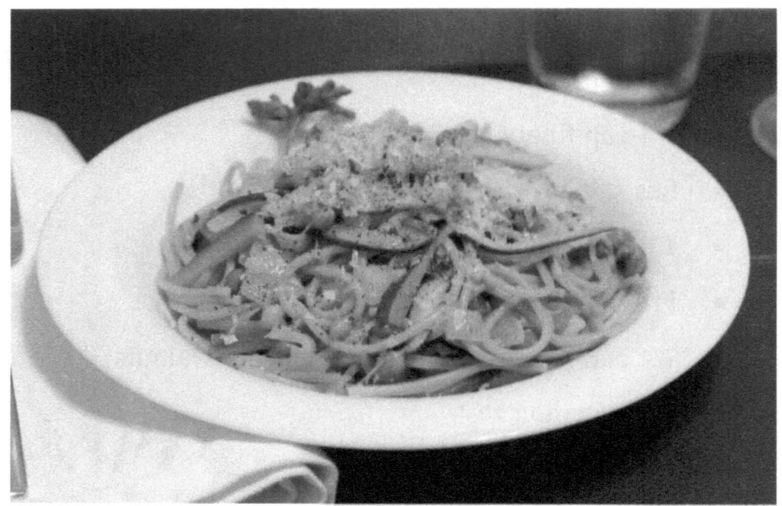

When you roast vegetables in olive oil quickly before you toss them with penne, they benefit from the taste upgrade. This recipe does not include any cream. It thrives on the freshest flavors of lemon, olive oil and balsamic vinegar.

Makes: 6 servings

Prep: 10 mins

Cook: 25 mins

Ingredients:

- 1 x 12-oz. pkg. of penne pasta
- 1 chopped squash, yellow
- 1 chopped zucchini
- 1 matchstick-cut carrot
- 1/2 matchstick-cut bell pepper, red
- 1/2 pint of tomatoes, grape
- 1 cup of trimmed, cut green beans, fresh
- 5 trimmed, sliced asparagus spears
- 1/4 cup of oil, olive
- 1 tbsp. of seasoning, Italian
- 1/2 tbsp. of lemon juice, fresh
- 1/4 tsp. of salt, kosher
- 1/4 tsp. of pepper, ground
- 1 tbsp. of butter, unsalted
- 1/4 sliced large onion, yellow
- 2 sliced garlic cloves
- 2 tsp. of lemon zest, fresh
- 1/3 cup of chopped basil leaves, fresh
- 1/3 cup of chopped parsley, fresh
- 3 tbsp. of vinegar, balsamic
- 1/2 cup of Romano cheese, grated

Directions:

Preheat the oven to 450F. Line cookie sheet with foil.

Bring pot of salted water to boil. Add pasta. Cook till firm yet tender to bite, about 10-12 minutes and drain.

Toss the squash, carrot, zucchini, tomatoes, bell pepper, asparagus and green beans together in bowl with 2 tbsp. oil and kosher salt, ground pepper, Italian seasoning and lemon juice. Arrange the veggies on baking sheet.

Roast the vegetables in 450F oven till they are tender, 12-15 minutes.

Heat the rest of the oil and the butter in large sized skillet. Cook the garlic and onion in the hot oil till they are tender, or five to seven minutes.

Mix the cooked pasta with vinegar, parsley, basil and lemon zest into onion mixture. Toss gently. Cook till heated fully through, about three to five minutes. Remove from the heat. Transfer to large sized bowl. Toss with the roasted veggies. Sprinkle with the Romano cheese and serve.

Chocolate Chia Pudding

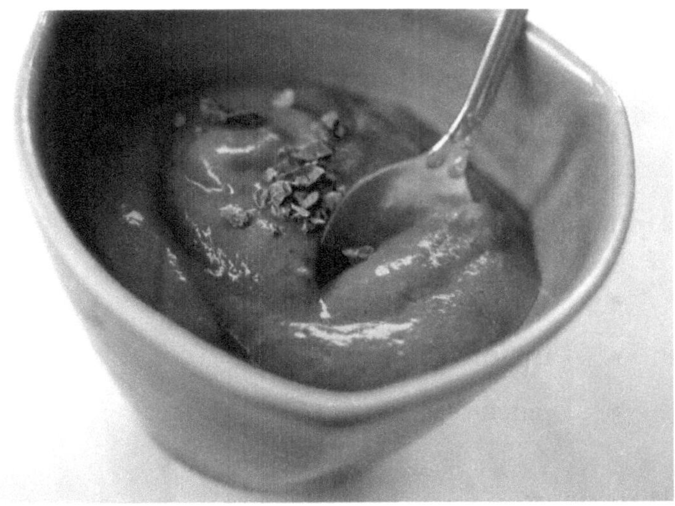

This pudding is lovely, sweet, creamy and rich – and SO delicious. The chia seeds are quite gut-friendly, and they give you a gentle fiber source that feeds the good bacteria in your digestive tract.

Makes: 2 servings

Prep: 2 hrs.

Cook: -

Ingredients:

- 2 cups of milk, non-dairy (like coconut or almond)
- 1 to 2 tbsp. of maple syrup +/- as desired
- 4 to 6 tbsp. of cocoa
- 1/2 cup of chia seeds

Optional add-ins:

- Sliced bananas or other sliced fruits
- 1 tsp. of vanilla, pure
- 1 pinch sea salt

Directions:

Mix all ingredients but chia seeds in blender. Blend till cocoa has been thoroughly mixed.

Taste and adjust as desired. Pour liquid into serving bowl. Add chia.

Allow bowl to set and stir it occasionally till it has set (this takes several hours). Serve.

Blueberry and Citrus Breakfast Parfait

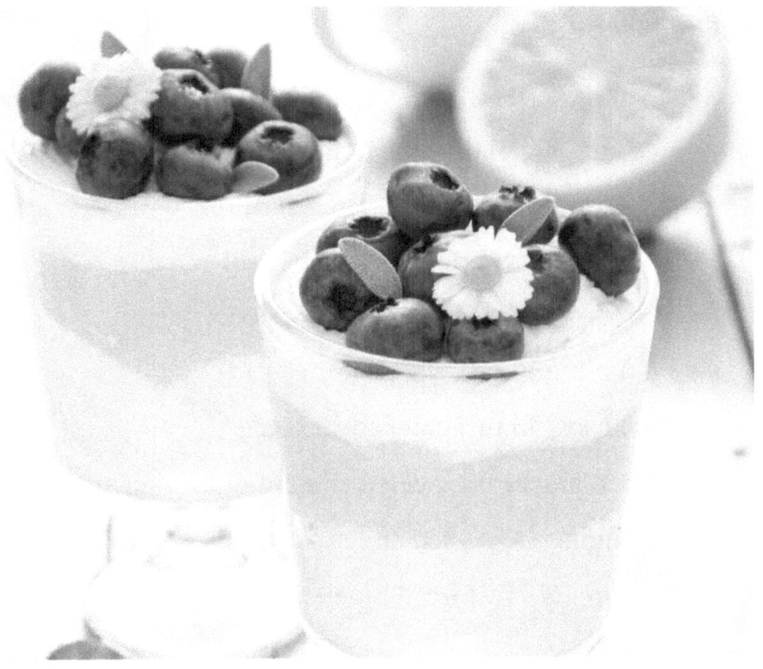

Parfaits are a simple yet visually pleasing breakfast option. Best of all, you can pack them full of your favorite fruits. Here we've added tangy citrus and antioxidant-loaded blueberries to a crunchy walnut, flax and wheat germ mix. Top it with some yogurt and you will definitely be starting your day off right!

Makes: 4 servings

Prep: 15 mins

Cook: -

Ingredients:

- 3 cups (710 ml) plain nonfat all-natural Greek yogurt or strained plain soy yogurt
- 1 Tbsp. (15 ml) pure maple syrup
- ½ tsp (2.5 ml) pure vanilla extract
- ½ cup (120 ml) walnuts, chopped
- 2 Tbsp. (30 ml) wheat germ
- 2 Tbsp. (30 ml) cracked flaxseed
- 1 red grapefruit, peeled and cut into small slices
- 1 Minneola, peeled and cut into small slices
- 1 cup (240 ml) fresh blueberries

Directions:

Stir together the yogurt, maple syrup and vanilla.

In four parfait glasses, pour in some of the yogurt mixture. Then sprinkle in some of the walnuts, wheat germ and flaxseeds, and then add some of the grapefruit, Minneola and blueberries.

Repeat until all of the remaining ingredients are used.

Maple & Turmeric Gelato

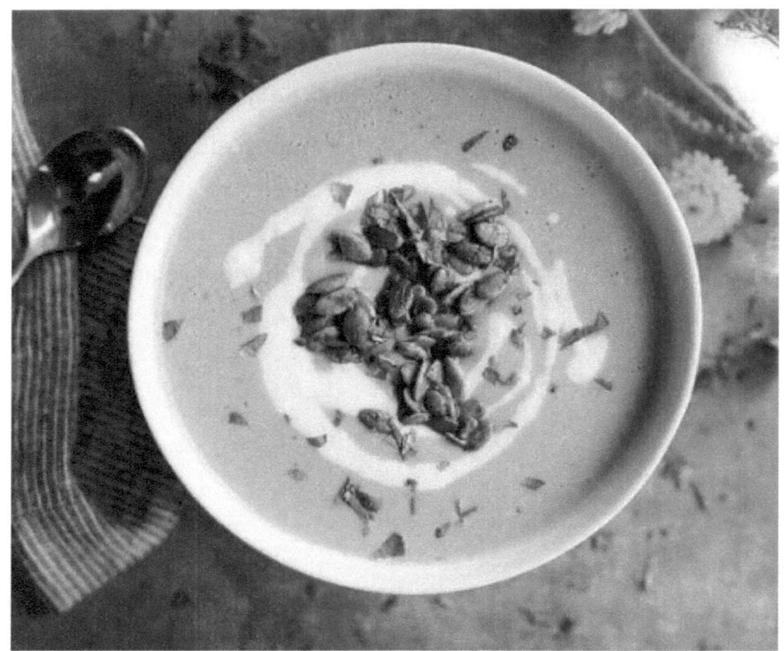

This gelato is made with maple syrup, turmeric and coconut milk. It's a vegan dessert choice and gives you a sweet summertime dessert without using any refined sugar.

Makes: 4 servings

Prep: 25 mins

Cook: -

Ingredients:

- 2 tsp. of coconut oil, refined
- 2 tsp. of powdered turmeric
- 3/4 cup of soaked, drained cashews
- 1 can of milk, coconut
- 1/3 cup of syrup, maple
- 1 tsp. of vanilla extract, pure
- 1 scraped vanilla bean
- 1 pinch of salt, sea

Directions:

Steep the turmeric in warmed coconut oil for eight to 10 minutes.

Place the coconut milk, cashews, syrup, coconut oil, vanilla bean, vanilla extract and sea salt in food processor. Blend till you have a smooth texture.

Churn the mixture in ice cream maker for 18-20 minutes, or till the consistency is soft serve. Transfer to the freezer and firm it up. Serve.

Acai Blueberry No-Churn Ice Cream

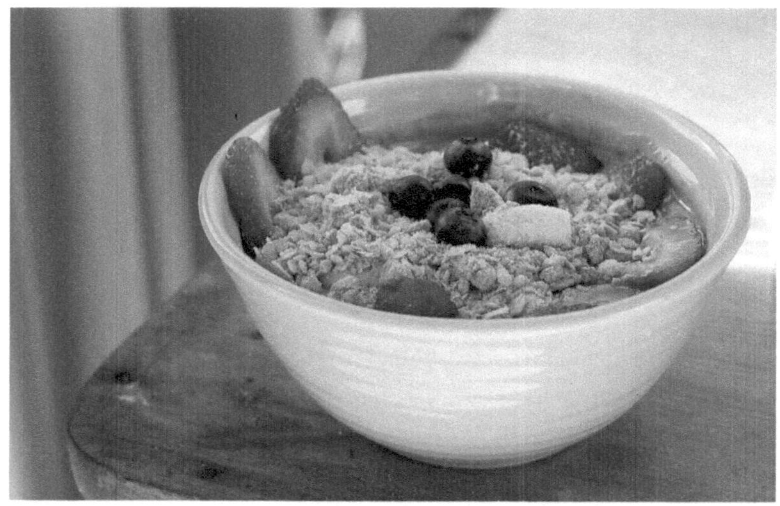

This Acai and blueberry ice cream needs no churning, and it bursts forth with the sweet taste of coconut and blueberries. It's healthier than ice cream and easier to make, too.

Makes: 8 servings

Prep: 6 hrs.

Cook: 10 mins

Ingredients:

- 1 pint of blueberries, fresh
- 1 pkt. of acai, frozen
- 1 can of coconut milk, full fat
- 1 tsp. of xanthan gum
- 1/3 cup of syrup, maple
- 1 tsp. of vanilla extract, pure

Directions:

Add all the ingredients to food processor. Blend till creamy and smooth.

Pour the ingredients in loaf pan. Cover with aluminum foil. Freeze till firm, four to five hours if you like soft serve and five to six hours for ice cream. Thaw for five to 10 minutes and serve.

Avocado Coconut Soup

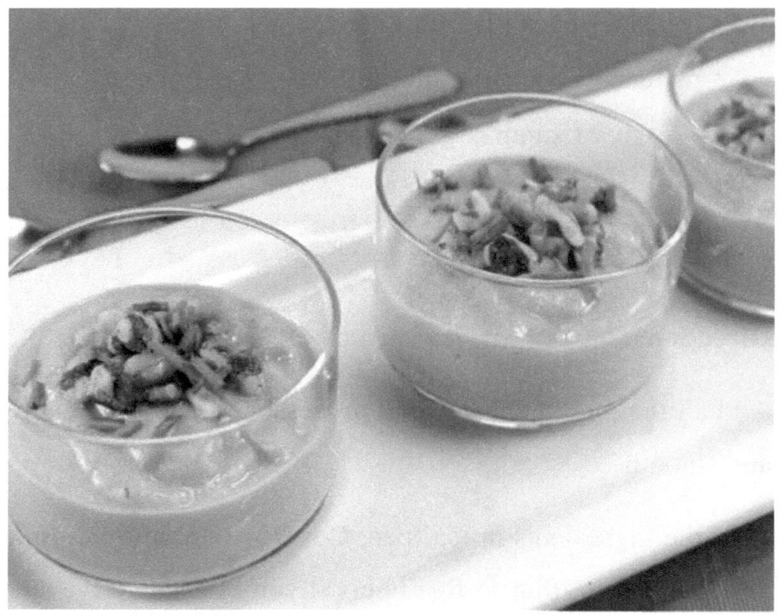

Avocado lends this soup a creamy texture, while coconut milk gives it a fresh and tropical flavor.

Makes: 4 servings

Prep: 2 hrs. + 5 mins

Cook: -

Ingredients:

- 1 1/2 cups coconut milk
- 1 1/2 cups water
- 2 ripe large avocados
- 1/4 cup packed fresh basil
- Juice of 1 lime
- 1 jalapeño chili pepper, seeded and minced
- 1/4 tsp. sea salt
- 1/4 tsp. freshly ground pepper, preferably white
- Grated zest of 1 lime

Directions:

Place all of the shown ingredients except the lime zest in a blender or food processor container and blend until smooth. If the mixture is too thick, simply blend in more coconut milk or water.

Pour the mixture into a container with a tight-fitting lid and refrigerate for at least 2 hours.

Garnish with lime zest when serving.

Quinoa Porridge with Walnut Cream

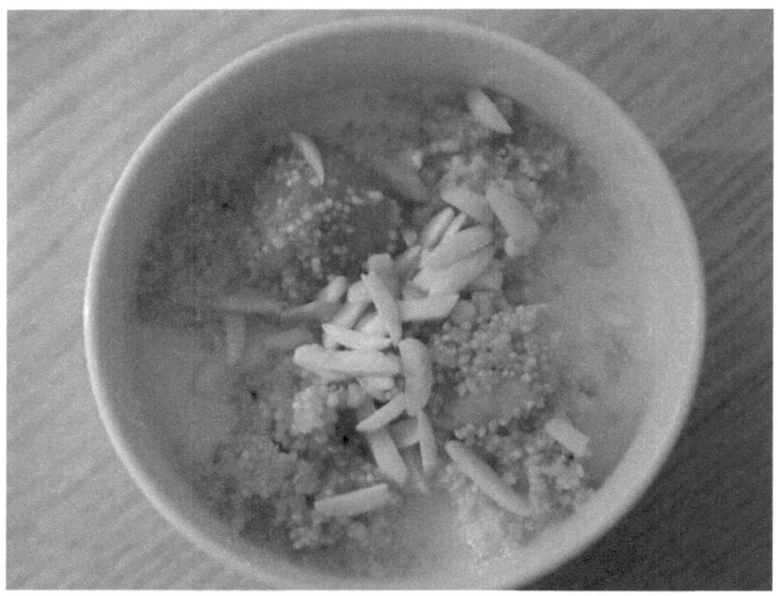

Protein is really important for staying strong during and after treatment, and quinoa is an excellent vegetable protein source. If you're a fan of oatmeal, millet, or buckwheat, you'll find that the slightly nutty, somewhat crunchy taste and texture of quinoa is right in your wheelhouse.

Makes: 6 servings

Prep: 10 mins

Cook: 20 mins

Ingredients:

- Walnut cream
- 1 cup walnuts
- 1 cup water
- 1 tsp. maple syrup
- 1 tsp. freshly squeezed lemon juice

Quinoa:

- ½ tsp. sea salt
- 2 cups water
- 1 cup quinoa
- 2 tbsp. of freshly squeezed orange juice
- ¼ tsp. sea salt
- 1 tbsp. maple syrup
- ⅛ tsp. ground nutmeg
- ½ tsp. ground ginger
- ¾ cup toasted coarsely chopped walnuts
- 1½ to 2 cups fresh blueberries, blackberries, raspberries
- 1 tsp. of ground cinnamon

Directions:

To make the walnut cream, place the walnuts in a bowl, put water to cover, and let stand overnight.

Preheat the oven to 350°F. Drain the walnuts well & spread on a baking pan. Toast for 8-10 mins or until they're lightly browned and aromatic, then cool completely.

Put the toasted walnuts, the lemon juice, 1 cup water, maple syrup, and salt in a blender. Blend on high speed until creamy & smooth, 1 to 2 mins. Move the cream to a bowl or jar.

For quinoa, rinse it in a strainer and drain it well. In a medium pan, bring the salt, quinoa, and water to boil over high. Lower to low, & then cover & simmer for about 15 minutes. Move aside off the heat to cool for a few minutes, then fluff with fork.

When you are ready to serve, stir ½ cup of the prepared walnut cream and the cinnamon, ginger, maple syrup, nutmeg, and orange juice into the cooked quinoa. Serve in bowls, & top with a spoonful of the walnut cream, some blueberries, & a sprinkling of toasted walnuts.

Roasted Kale

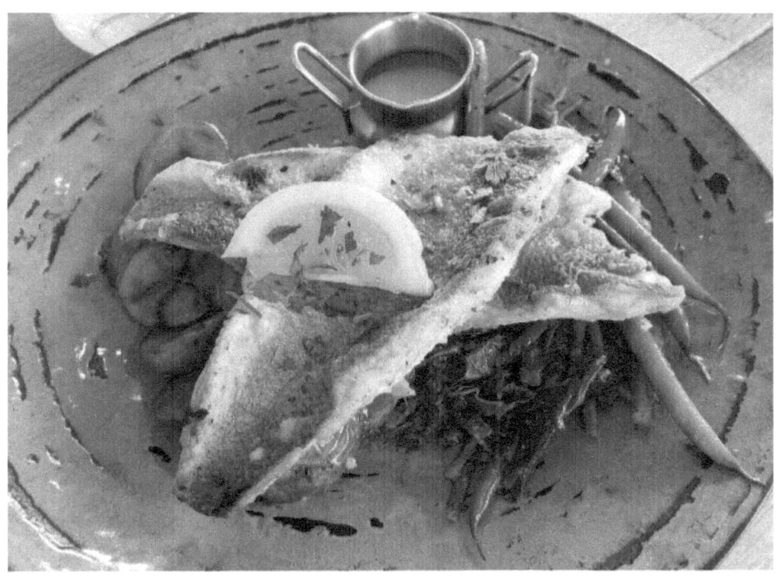

Kale is packed full of healthy phytonutrients.

Makes: 2 servings

Prep: 10 mins

Cook: 15 mins

Ingredients:

- 6 cups kale
- 1 tbsp. olive oil
- 1 tsp. garlic powder
- 1 tsp. sea salt

Directions:

Preheat oven to 375°F.

Wash & trim kale by pulling leaves off the tough stems or running a sharp knife down the length of the stem.

Place leaves in a medium-size bowl; toss with olive oil and garlic powder.

Roast for 5 minutes; turn kale over and roast another 7–10 minutes, until the kale turns brown and it becomes paper thin and brittle.

Remove from oven and sprinkle with salt. Serve immediately.

Lemony Apple Fennel Salad

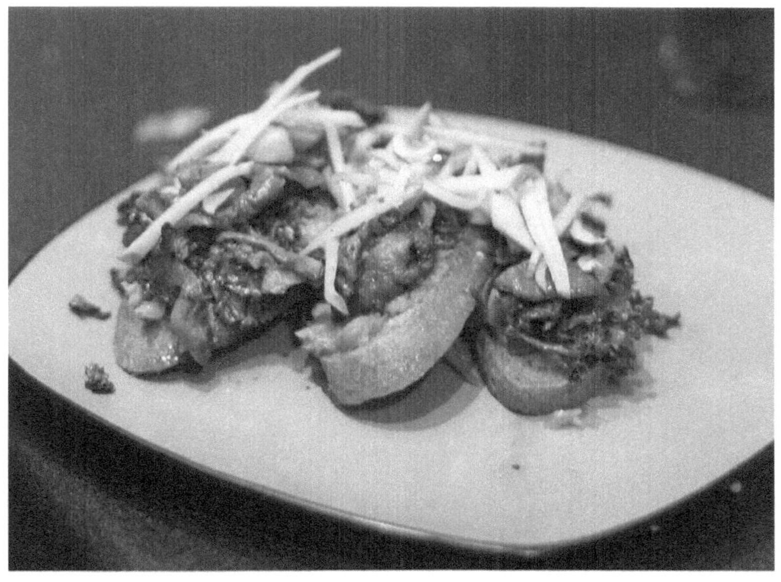

c

With its slight licorice flavor and crunchy texture, fennel is wonderful served raw in salads and it tastes even better combined with apples, arugula and zucchini.

Makes: 4 servings

Prep: 10 mins

Cook: -

Ingredients:

For the salad:

- 1 fennel bulb, thinly sliced
- 2 cups packed arugula
- 1/4 cup chopped fresh mint (optional)
- 2 medium apples, thinly sliced
- 1 medium zucchini, shredded (about 1 cup)

For the dressing:

- 3 tbsp. olive oil
- 1 tbsp. honey
- Juice of 1/2 lemon
- 1 tsp. grated lemon zest
- 1 clove garlic, minced
- 1/4 tsp. sea salt
- 1/4 tsp. freshly ground black pepper

Directions:

For salad: In a bowl, combine together the fennel, apple, arugula, zucchini, and mint if using.

For dressing: In a bowl, combine together the olive oil, honey, lemon juice, lemon zest, garlic, salt, & pepper.

Toss and serve.

Ginger and Lemon Drink

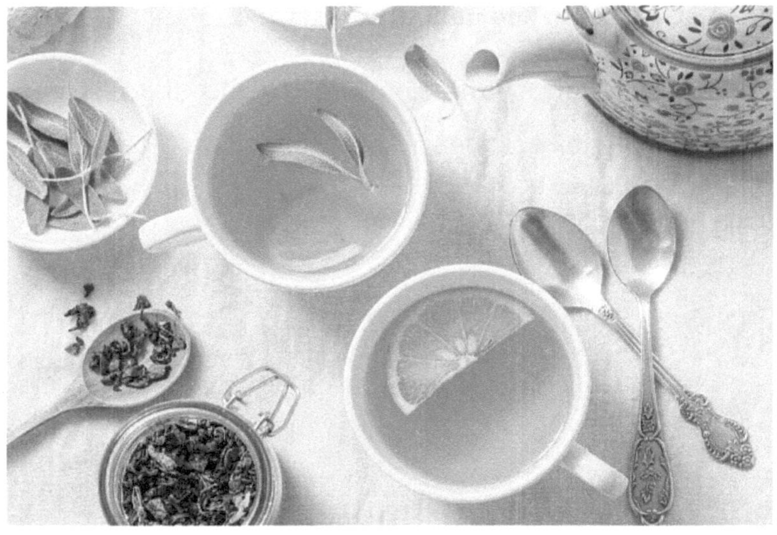

A warm, healing ginger lemon drink with turmeric and honey.

Makes: 3 servings

Prep: 30 mins

Cook: 5 mins

Ingredients:

- 1 piece Lemon, organic, sliced
- 1/8 tsp Turmeric, ground
- 2 ½ cups Water, boiling
- 1 piece Ginger, fresh, 1-inch, peeled, and sliced
- 2 tsp. Honey

Directions:

Pour water into a pot and heat on medium-high. Once boiling, immediately turn off the heat.

Stir in the turmeric, ginger, and lemon.

Let it steep for 1/2 an hour.

Strain before serving.

Enjoy.

Ginger-Turmeric Cauliflower

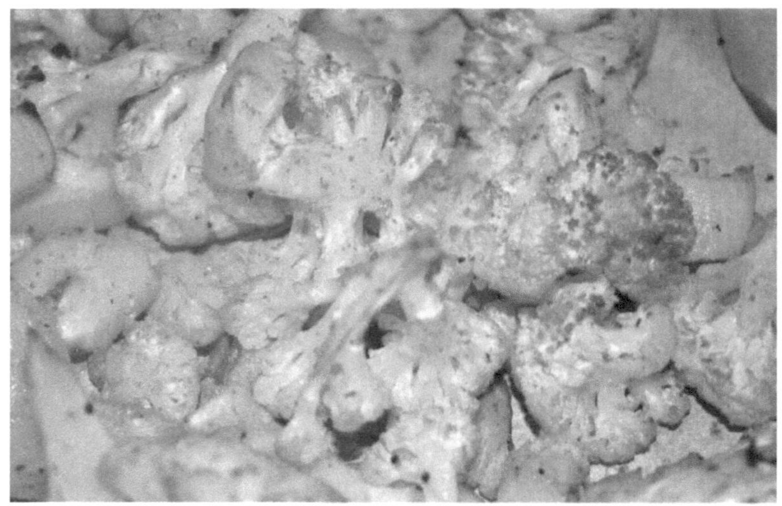

Ginger turmeric cauliflower with avocado oil and ginger. Turmeric is said to help relieve GERD symptoms.

Makes: 6 servings

Prep: 10 mins

Cook: 25 mins

Ingredients:

- 1/2 tsp. Red pepper flakes
- 1/4 cup Avocado oil
- 1 ½ tsp. Cumin, ground
- 2 tbsp. Parsley, flat leaf, Italian, chopped
- 2 tsp. Turmeric, ground
- 3/4 tsp. Black pepper, freshly ground
- 2 pieces Cauliflower heads
- 2 tbsp. Lemon juice, freshly squeezed
- 2 tsp. Ginger, ground
- 1 ½ tsp. Sea salt
- 2 tbsp. Pomegranate arils

Directions:

Set the oven at 400 degrees Fahrenheit to preheat.

Use parchment paper to line a large baking sheet. Lightly coat with avocado oil and set aside.

After washing and separating the cauliflower into florets, place inside a large bowl.

Meanwhile, whisk the lemon juice, spices, and oil in a small bowl. Add to the cauliflower and toss until well-combined.

Transfer the seasoned cauliflower onto the lined sheet. Roast in the oven for about twenty to twenty-five minutes or until lightly browned.

Allow to cool before serving garnished with pomegranate arils and chopped parsley.

Overnight Oats

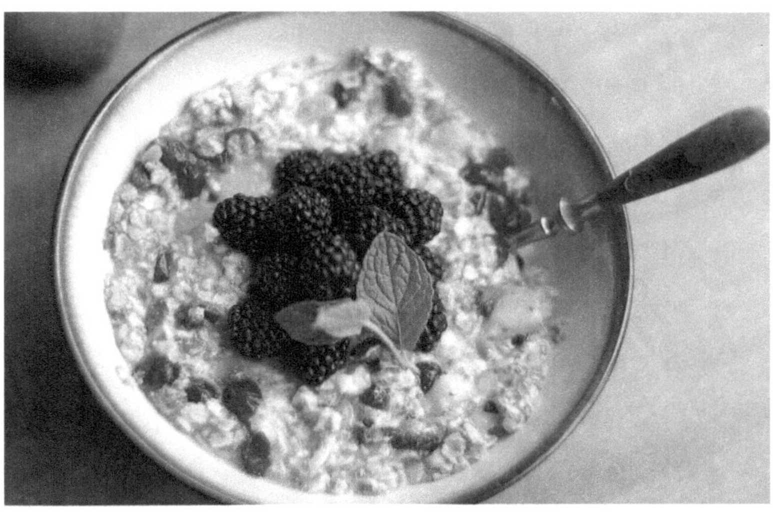

In our busy world, few people have time to cook up hearty steel-cut oats in the morning. Thankfully, soaking steel-cut oats overnight softens their texture so they can be enjoyed uncooked. The result is a deliciously chewy and ¬filling breakfast cereal.

Makes: 4 servings

Prep: 5 mins plus overnight

Cook: -

Ingredients:

- 2 cups steel-cut oats
- ½ cup almond flour
- 3 tbsp. chia seeds
- 2 tbsp. pure maple syrup
- 1 tsp. vanilla extract
- 1 tsp. ground cinnamon
- ½ tsp. ground nutmeg
- 2 cups milk
- 1/2 cup chopped nuts
- 1 cup berries of choice

Directions:

Add all of the ingredients in a large container and stir until well combined. Cover and refrigerate overnight.

Pumpkin Oat Bars

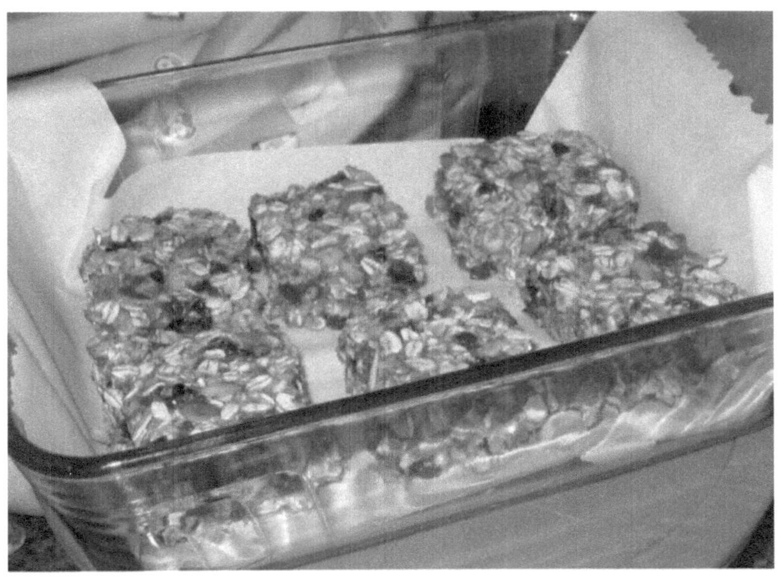

Here's a fresh and delicious recipe to add some flair to snack time.

Makes: 4 servings

Prep: 10 mins plus 1 hr.

Cook: -

Ingredients:

- 3/4 cup unsalted natural peanut butter or other nut butter of choice
- 3/4 cup canned pumpkin puree
- 2 tbsp. molasses
- 2 cups granola of choice, plus more for topping
- ½ cup oat bran
- ½ cup non-instant milk powder
- ½ tsp. ground cinnamon
- 1/3 cup dried currants
- ½ tsp. ground ginger
- ¼ tsp. ground cloves
- Pinch of sea salt

Directions:

Prepare an 8X8 inch pan with paper.

Place the peanut butter, pumpkin and molasses in a large bowl and mix until well combined. Add in the remaining ingredients & mix until everything is moist. The mixture should be thick.

Place the mixture the prepared pan and spread it out until you have an even thickness of about 1/2 inch. Sprinkle some additional granola on top and press down lightly. Place in the freezer for about 1 hr.

Slice into bars and store in an airtight container in the refrigerator.

Blueberry Pie Protein Drink

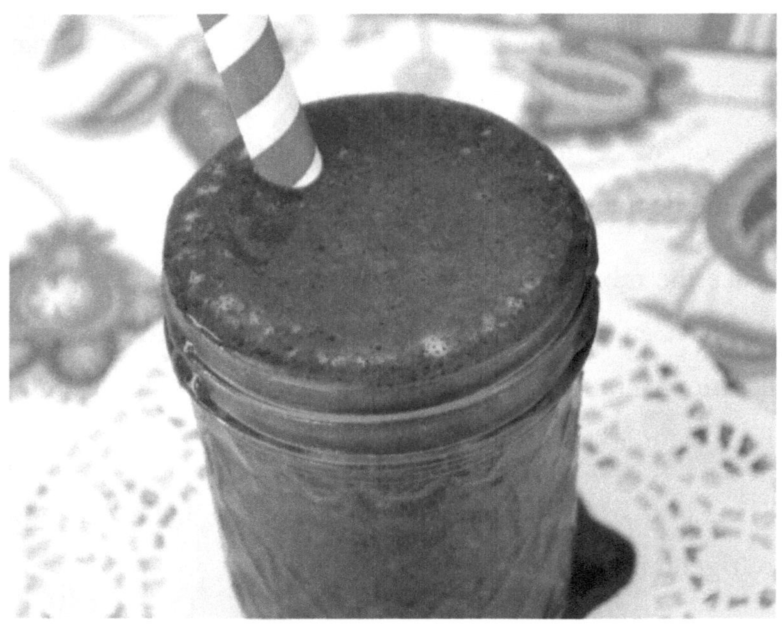

Delicious protein filled blueberry pie drink. Perfect for on-the-go breakfast that's easy on the stomach!

Makes: 1 serving

Prep: 5 mins

Cook: -

Ingredients:

- ½ cup frozen unsweetened wild blueberries
- Juice of ½ lemon
- 1 scoop vanilla protein powder
- ½ cup water
- ½ cup ice

Directions:

Blend all ingredients until thoroughly combined.

Braised Leeks with Herbs

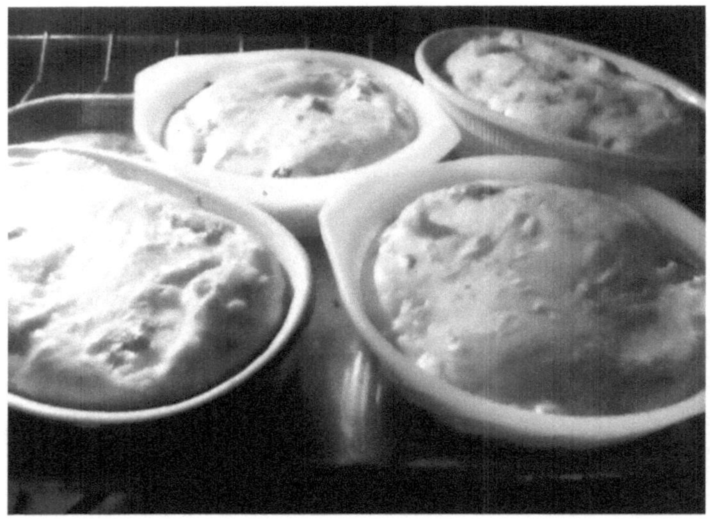

When you cook this healthy dish in your oven, it develops a pleasing, silky texture. The leeks are often served with fish or roast chicken.

Makes: 4 servings

Prep: 10 mins

Cook: 1 hr.

Ingredients:

- 4 leeks, large
- 3 tbsp. of oil, olive
- 1/2 tsp. of herbs de Provence – available at local markets or online
- 1/2 tsp. of pepper, ground
- 1/4 tsp. of salt, kosher

Directions:

Preheat the oven to 350F. Trim the dark green tops and roots from the leeks. Leave five to eight inches of light green and white parts. Slice leeks lengthways in halves. Rinse thoroughly, and remove grit, if any. Pat the leeks dry.

Nestle leeks in one layer. They can be laid on the sides if you need to, in 13x9" baking dish. Drizzle leeks with oil. Use herbs de Provence, kosher salt and ground pepper to sprinkle.

Cover baking dish with aluminum foil. Bake till quite tender, for 50 minutes to an hour. Uncover dish. Continue to bake till browned lightly, or 8-10 more minutes. Serve.

Marinated Mushroom Salad

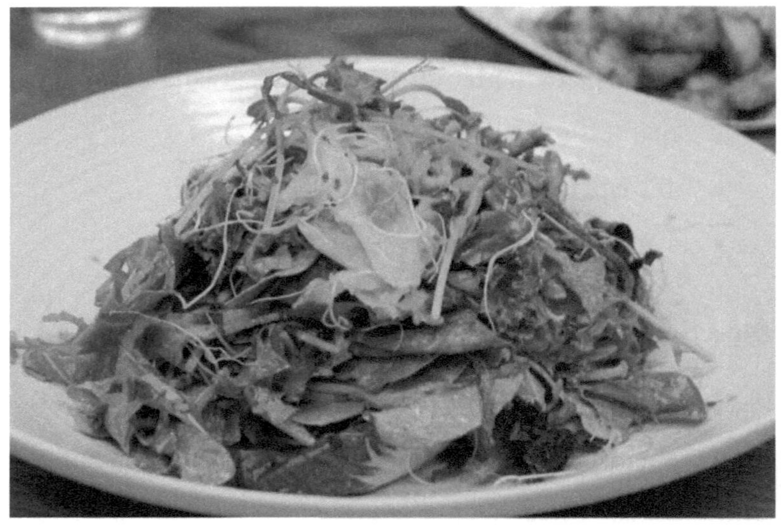

A delicious marinated mushroom salad with cherry tomatoes, thyme and walnuts.

Makes: 4 servings

Prep: 10 mins plus chilling time

Cook: -

Ingredients:

- 4 cups mushrooms, thinly sliced
- 1 ½ cups cherry tomatoes, sliced in half
- 4 tbsp. extra virgin olive oil
- 3 tbsp. white wine or 2 tbsp. white wine vinegar
- 1 clove garlic, minced
- 2 tsp. Dijon mustard
- 2 tsp. fresh thyme
- 1 tsp. fennel seeds (optional)
- 1/2 tsp. sea salt
- 1/4 tsp. freshly ground black pepper
- 1/3 cup coarsely chopped at-leaf parsley
- 2 cups spinach
- 1/3 cup chopped walnuts, for garnish
- 4 tbsp. grated Parmesan or Gruyere cheese, for garnish
- Truffle oil, for garnish (optional)

Directions:

In a bowl, combine the mushrooms and tomatoes. In a separate bowl, whisk together the oil, wine or vinegar, garlic, mustard, thyme, fennel seeds if using, salt and black pepper.

Add the oil mix to the mushrooms and tomatoes and toss to coat. Let it marinate in the refrigerator for at least 2 hours or up to overnight, stirring a couple of times.

Mix the parsley into the mushroom mixture. Arrange the spinach on serving plates and top with mushroom salad. Garnish with walnuts, grated cheese, and truffle oil if desired.

Serve.

Coconut Pecan Granola

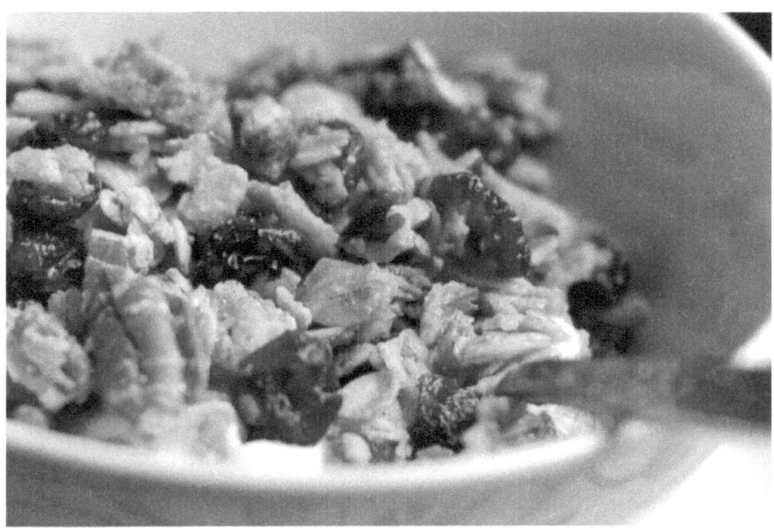

Sprinkle this delicious granola on your oatmeal or on top of your smoothie bowls.

Makes: 5 cups

Prep: 10 mins

Cook: 25 mins

Ingredients:

- 2 cups rolled oats
- ½ cup flaked coconut
- ½ cup pecans, chopped
- 3 tbsp. honey

Directions:

Preheat the oven to 300°F.

Combine together the oats, coconut, pecan, and honey in a large baking pan.

Bake or 15 minutes. Remove and stir and then bake for 10 minutes more. Cool.

Store granola in an air-tight container.

Conclusion

There you have it! 30 delicious and nutritious recipes that help keep GERD at bay! Make sure to try out all of the recipes in the book and be if you love them (we hope you do), be sure to share them with your friends and family!

About the Author

Allie Allen developed her passion for the culinary arts at the tender age of five when she would help her mother cook for their large family of 8. Even back then, her family knew this would be more than a hobby for the young Allie and when she graduated from high school, she applied to cooking school in London. It had always been a dream of the young chef to study with some of Europe's best and she made it happen by attending the Chef Academy of London.

After graduation, Allie decided to bring her skills back to North America and open up her own restaurant. After 10 successful years as head chef and owner, she decided to sell her business and pursue other career avenues. This monumental decision led Allie to her true calling, teaching. She also started to write e-books for her students to study at home for practice. She is now the proud author of several e-books and gives private and semi-private cooking lessons to a range of students at all levels of experience.

Stay tuned for more from this dynamic chef and teacher when she releases more informative e-books on cooking and baking in the near future. Her work is infused with stores and anecdotes you will love!

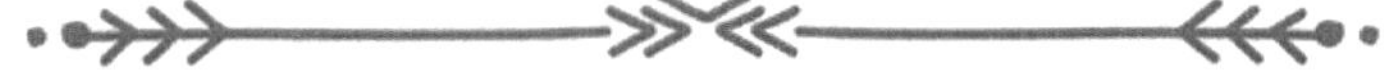

Author's Afterthoughts

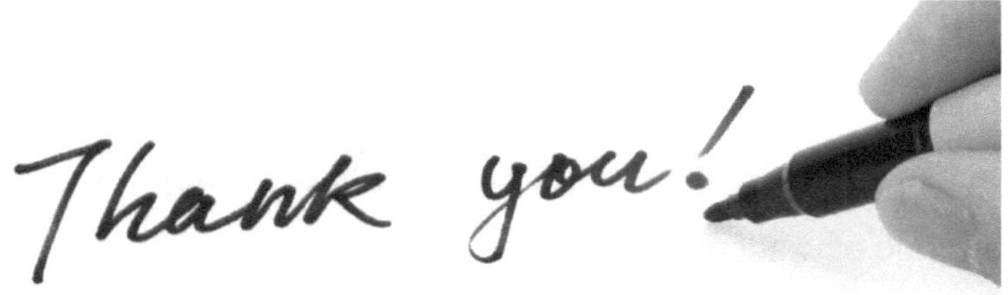

I can't tell you how grateful I am that you decided to read my book. My most heartfelt thanks that you took time out of your life to choose my work and I hope you find benefit within these pages.

There are so many books available today that offer similar content so that makes it even more humbling that you decided to buying mine.

Tell me what you thought! I am eager to hear your opinion and ideas on what you read as are others who are looking for a good book to buy. Leave a review on Amazon.com so others can benefit from your wisdom!

With much thanks,

Allie Allen

www.ingramcontent.com/pod-product-compliance
Lightning Source LLC
Chambersburg PA
CBHW031152250726
48655CB00002B/936